THAI PALEO

Authentic Recipes Made Easy

Disclaimer

Contents

Summary

Thai cuisine consists of a wide range of delicious recipes. Being one of the richest cuisines, Thai recipes are not only famous in Asia, but enjoyed all across the world. However, calorie conscious people cannot treat themselves with the enthralling taste of creamy Thai soups and high calorie diet. One way to do so is replace high carbs or fatty ingredients with some other healthy elements.

Here in this eBook you can find:

- The perfect blend of Paleo and Thai dishes.
- You can find 50 easy-to-cook recipes, which are not only mouthwatering, but will also keep you healthy, strong and lean.
- Unlike other recipe books which only focus on taste, this eBook contains recipes which will allow you to enjoy pure Thai cuisine but in a healthy way.

Thai-Paleo recipes in this eBook have preserved the original taste of Thai food. Also in this eBook you will find:

- Nutritional value.
- Serving size.
- And preparation time of every recipe, thus allowing you to keep a check on your daily calorie count.

If you want to enthrall your taste buds with delicious Paleo-Thai recipes and reap countless health benefits, then keep exploring this eBook!

Paleo-Thai Appetizers

A Thai cuisine has a wide assortment of easy-to-cook and healthy appetizers. The addition of Paleo ingredients has doubled the health benefits of these appetizers. Have a peek at some of these amazing recipes!

Chicken Soup

This is probably the healthiest appetizers of all times. You can add Paleo spices to add plain Thai chicken soup and enjoy tasty soup within no time. You can serve this appetizer with roasted chicken to complete the platter!

Ingredients

For Broth

1 ½ chicken carcass

Lemongrass (2 pieces), finely chopped

Chili powder, ½ tbsp

Lime juice, 1 tbsp

2 medium sized onions, roughly chopped

5 large garlic cloves, peeled and minced

½ piece ginger, finely chopped

For Soup

Coconut aminos, 2 tbsp

Lime juice, 1 ½ tbsp

3 Spring onions (only green part), finely chopped

½ ginger, finely chopped

Organic coconut milk, 70 ml

Kelp noodles, half packet (almost 50g)

Sea salt, to taste

Directions

Start with heat the chicken carcass in a large pan.

Add almost 1 liter of distilled water and heat the carcass for an hour.

You might need to add water from time to time.

Drain the broth in a bowl.

Only use 150ml of chicken broth for the soup and refrigerate the rest.

Pour the drained broth in a small pan and heat with all the ingredients (for broth) on small flame.

Meanwhile cook the kelp noodles and add coconut milk, amino sauce and rest of the ingredients.

Don't let the noodles mixture come to boil.

Mix the noodles soup with chicken broth and enjoy warm!

Servings

2 persons

Preparation Time

1 hour 30 minutes

Nutritional Facts

Calories	Carbs	Fat	Protein
282.7	48.9g	8.7g	6.9g

Cashew Sauce

Peanut sauce is one of the most famous appetizers of Thai cuisine. However, replacing peanuts with cashews not only changes the taste of this appetizer, but also makes it healthier than ever. Do try this easy-to-make Paleo-Thai Cashew sauce and experience the difference.

Ingredients

Cashew (unsalted), 2 cups

3 large garlic cloves peeled and mince

Distilled water, 4 tbsp

Sea salt, to taste

Organic coconut milk, 1 cup

Lime juice, 4 tbsp

Shredded salmon, 1 cup

Chili powder (organic), to taste

Paprika (optional), a pinch

Directions

In a pan, heat coconut milk on medium flame and add shredded fish to it.

Add cashew to the mixture and stir well.

After 5 minutes, add the rest of the ingredients and mix well.

Turn off the flame and dish out the sauce.

Enjoy with crackers or cutlets.

Servings

16 persons

Preparation Time

20 minutes

Nutritional Facts

Calories	Carbs	Fat	Protein
160	5.7g	13.4g	6.6g

Thai Spring Fruits Salsa

Shallow fried spring fruits, can serve the purpose of an appetizer or provide the nutrition of complete mean to those who prefer low carbs diet. It is probably one of the easiest appetizers which can be prepared from few ingredients.

Ingredients

Finely diced mango, 1 cup

Cucumber (peeled and chopped), 1 cup

Strawberries (fresh and sliced), 1 cup

Cantaloupe (chopped), 1 cup

Spring onion (both parts), ½ cup finely chopped

Lime juice, 2 ½ tbsp

Raw honey, 1 tbsp

Mind leaves, chopped

Finely grounded pepper, ½ tsp

Basil (fresh), 1 ½ tbsp

Sea salt, ½ tsp

Note: You can add any fruit of your choice.

Directions

In a large bowl toss all the raw fruits together.

Add rest of the ingredients and mix together.

Enjoy!

Servings

6 persons

Preparation Time

15 minutes

Nutritional Facts

Calories	Carbs	Fat	Protein
45	11g	0g	0.5g

Want some spicy appetizer? Here you go! Try this unique combination of Paleo crackers with organic vegetables and treat you taste buds.

Ingredients

Tahini paste, 4 tbsp

Organic Mustard, 1 tbsp

Coconut flour, 3 tbsp

Coconut oil, 1 tbsp

1 large (organic) egg

4 tomatoes (peeled and unseeded), plumed

5 shallots, peeled and roughly chopped

Lime juice (for vegetables), 10 tsp

Directions

Preheat the oven to 340oF.

In a bowl, mix egg, coconut flour and coconut oil together.

Add mustard to the batter and fold.

Make small balls of the batter and gently flatten with your hands.

Bake these crackers for 5 minutes.

Meanwhile mix plumed tomatoes, garlic and shallots in another bowl.

Add a pinch of coconut oil and toss vegetables together.

Sprinkle sea salt and pepper and mix well.

Enjoy with freshly baked crackers.

Servings

2 persons

Preparation Time

20 minutes

Nutritional Facts

Calories	Carbs	Fat	Protein
300	42g	14g	8g

Shrimps with Coconut Dipping

Thai appetizers list cannot be completed without dipped shrimps. Here is a slightly modified version of shrimps with peanut sauce. The Paleo version has replaced peanut sauce with coconut dipping. Try this variation of dipped shrimps!

Ingredients

Coconut Aminos, approximately 10ounces

Coconut milk (organic), 1 cup

Paprika, 1 tsp

Black pepper (freshly grounded). 1 tsp

Sea salt, to taste

Grass fed butter, 1 tbsp

Frozen shrimps, 1 medium packet

Directions

Heat the frozen shrimps (according to the packet directions)

In a small pan, heat coconut milk, grass fed butter, salt, paprika and pepper over a medium flame.

Keep stirring the mixture to combine all the ingredients well.

Pour the coconut milk in a bowl and add coconut aminos sauce in it.

Enjoy shrimps with coconut dipping.

Servings

5 persons

Preparation Time

30 minutes

Nutritional Facts

Calories	Carbs	Fat	Protein
130	10g	9g	2g

Paleo-Thai Breakfast Recipes

Thai Spinach Wraps

This breakfast is perfect for those who want to shed extra pounds. This easy-to-cook dish is a unique blend of crispy vegetables, wrapped in spinach leaves.

Ingredients

Organic fish sauce, a dash

2 fresh limes, chopped and segmented

Half ginger, finely chopped

Maple syrup, 1 tsp

1 shallot, chopped

Coriander leaves, 2 tbsp

Spinach leaves 10-12

Chili powder, 1 tsp

Sea salt, according to taste

Directions

In a small bowl, toss fresh lime, chopped shallot, and ginger and coriander together.

Sprinkle chili powder and salt and mix well.

Season the mixture with fish sauce and maple syrup.

In a flat tray, spread spinach leaves.

Put a small amount of seasoned mixture in a very leave and roll.

Enjoy crispy spinach wraps.

Servings

4 persons

Preparation Time

10 minutes

Nutritional Facts

Calories	Carbs	Fat	Protein
36	2g	2g	2g

Red Chicken Cutlets

This dish is a lovely blend of vegetables and chicken for meat lovers. Enjoy the sizzling Thai taste in Paleo style.

Ingredients

2 chicken breast pieces (skinless), diced into large square chunks

Fish sauce, 2 tbsp

Tomato paste, 2 tbsp

Organic coconut milk, 2 ½ tbsp

1 fresh lemon, for serving

2 small red pepper, chopped

Red onion, peeled and chopped

Directions

Heat a large skillet over medium flame.

Meanwhile, start preparing for marinating paste in a large bowl.

Mix coconut milk with fish sauce and tomato paste.

Coat chicken pieces with the marinating paste and set aside.

Thread onion wedges and chicken chunks onto skewers and barbecue for 8-10 minutes.

Make sure that the chicken is juicy and tender.

Season with lemon juice and enjoy.

Servings

2 persons

Preparation Time

20 minutes

Nutritional Facts

Calories	Carbs	Fat	Protein
251	10g	8g	36g

Vegetable Thai Broth

Are you a soup lover? Then this dish is perfect for you! Cooked with in no time, this recipe is a unique blend of fish and vegetables.

Ingredients

Organic Thai curry (Paleo), 2 tbsp

6 large tomatoes, sliced into halves

Coconut oil, 1 tsp

Chinese cabbage head, ½

Coconut milk, 400ml

2 small carrots, finely chopped

Kelp noodles, 1 packet

Raw honey, 2 tsp

Lime juice, 4 tbsp

Coriander leaves, finely chopped

3 small spring onions, green and white part finely sliced

Directions

Heat coconut oil over small flame.

Add curry paste to the oil and heat for 1 minute.

Add vegetables, raw honey and coconut milk to the mixture and toss well.

Add boiled noodles to the mixture and simmer for 5 minutes.

Add lime juice to the mixture and mix well.

Turn off the flame and enjoy.

Servings

4 persons

Preparation Time

25 minutes

Nutritional Facts

Calories	Carbs	Fat	Protein
338	46g	5g	10g

Thai Green Soup

Green soup is a very healthy Thai breakfast and perfect for calorie conscious people!

Ingredients

Coconut oil, 2 ½ tbsp

1 large spring onion green part finely chopped and white part roughly diced

1 onion, peeled and roughly chopped

Chicken breast or thigh fillets, 500g chopped

Fish sauce, 2 1.2 tbsp

Chicken broth, 2l

Thai curry paste (green and Paleo), 1 small jar

Coconut milk, 1 can (400ml approx)

2 Capsicum (unseeded), squarely diced

Lime juice, ½ cup

Directions

In a large pan and heat coconut milk over small flame.

Add curry paste, chicken broth, chicken fillet and fish sauce to the milk and heat for 10minutes,

As the mixture starts simmering, add diced onions and capsicum and stir for 5 minutes.

Mean while blend the green part of spring onion with lemon juice in a food processor to form a green paste.

Add this paste to the coconut milk mixture and heat for few minutes.

Enjoy warm soup.

Servings

8 persons

Preparation Time

1 hour

Nutritional Facts

Calories	Carbs	Fat	Protein
262	8g	16g	23g

Thai Baked and Crumbed Chicken

Want to start your day with something crunchy? Then here is a perfect recipe for you. Easy-to-prepare baked chicken is not only healthy but also delicious!

Ingredients

1 butternut pumpkin, unseeded and roughly diced

Dried coconut, 1 tbsp

Coconut oil, 1 ½ tbsp

Fresh lime wedges, for serving

Coriander leaves, handful finely chopped

4 chicken breast pieces, skinless

Red Thai curry paste, 2 ½ tbsp

Tomato paste, 300g

1 egg, beaten

1 large sized eggplant, cubed

For Crumbs

Almond/coconut flour, ½ cup

Coconut flakes, ½ cup finely crushed

Sea salt, 1 tbsp

Lemon zest, 1 tsp

Garlic powder, 1 tsp

Pepper, 1 tbsp

Directions

In a small bowl combine all the ingredients for crumbs and set aside.

Preheat the oven to 200°C.

In a large tin bowl, toss eggplant with butternut squash.

Add coconut oil to it and roast for 30 minutes.

In a speared flat plate, mix crumbs mixture and dried coconut together.

Soak chicken breast pieces in beaten egg and coat with crumbs mixture.

Add curry and tomato paste to the roasted eggplant and mix well.

Toss crumbs coated chicken pieces with the vege mixtures.

Roast for 30 minutes.

Take out the chicken when tender and juicy.

Season with fresh lime juice and enjoy.

Servings

4 persons

Preparation Time

1 hr 15 minutes

Nutritional Facts

Calories	Carbs	Fat	Protein
414	32g	15g	38g

Thai Low Carbs Fish Broth

This is an extremely low calorie breakfast. You can also replace fish broth with chicken stock and enjoy Thai chicken broth.

Ingredients

Kelp noodles, 100g packet

Handful coriander leaves, finely chopped

Fish stock, 500ml

Raw prawns, 100g

Fish sauce, 1tbsp

Skinless fish (any Paleo), 200g

Directions

Boil noodles and drain with cold water.

Heat fish stock in a large pan over medium flame.

Add Thai curry and fish sauce and stir well.

Bring the mixture to simmer.

Meanwhile, dice the skinless fish in small cubes.

Add these cubes to the fish sauce mixture and cook for 5 minutes.

Add noodles and prawns to the mixture and stir for 2 minutes.

Turn off the flame and enjoy!

Servings

2 persons

Preparation Time

25 minutes

Nutritional Facts

Calories	Carbs	Fat	Protein
330	35g	4g	40g

Thai Skinny Burgers

This is a perfect recipe for kids. You can make these burgers with in no time and also enjoy them as snacks.

Ingredients for Filling

4 carrots, diced

Coconut oil, 1 tbsp

1 small sized gem lettuce

Minced meat (beef preferably), 500g

Chili paste, 2 ½ tbsp

2 red chilies, unseeded and chopped

Thai curry paste, 2 ½ tbsp

Lime juice, 2 tbsp

1 small coriander bunch, finely chopped

6 small spring onions, green and white part finely chopped

Ingredients for Paleo Buns

4 eggs

Coconut flour, 3 tbsp

Sea salt, a pinch

Coconut oil, 3 tbsp

Baking powder, 1 tbsp

Directions

For Buns

Preheat the oven to 360ºF.

Mean while, mix coconut flour, sea salt and baking powder together.

In another bowl whisk eggs and add coconut oil.

Mix the dry and wet mixture together and fold until combined well.

Pour the batter into a flat baking tray and bake for 10 minutes.

For Filling

Preheat oven to 200ºC.

Meanwhile start preparing for mince meat patties.

In a bowl mix curry paste, coriander leaves and spring onion.

Add minced meat to the paste and blend well.

Shape into patties.

Bake for 10 minutes.

Take out when tender and juicy.

Sandwich between toasted buns.

Enjoy with chili and fish sauce dipping.

Servings

4 persons

Preparation Time

50 minutes

Nutritional Facts

Calories	Carbs	Fat	Protein
700	82g	16g	46g

Thai Morning Squash

The unique blend of butternut squash and coconut milk can enthrall your taste buds. With a very few ingredients you can enjoy these mouthwatering dish.

Ingredients

1 large onion, peeled and finely chopped

1 coriander leaves bunch, picked

Organic coconut milk, 150ml

1 stalk of lemongrass, finely shredded

Lemon juice, 1 lime

Butternut squash, 1 ½ kg finely diced

Directions

In a large pan, shallow fry diced onions with lemongrass, until softened.

If the onion starts catching up, splash water.

Add butternut squash and stir.

Add approximately 1 liter water and cover the pan with a lid.

Leave for 10minutes, until the mixture starts simmering.

Add lemon juice, stir lightly and remove from the flame.

Add coconut milk to the mixture and blend well.

Enjoy with chili sauce,

Servings

4 persons

Preparation Time

20 minutes

Nutritional Facts

Calories	Carbs	Fat	Protein
161	23g	6g	4g

Lemon Grass Stew

Nothing can be more refreshing than the unique blend of beef and lemongrass. You can also replace beef with chicken or pork.

Ingredients

Beef (stewed), 250g diced into small cubes

Peeled ginger, 1 tbsp finely chopped

Coconut oil, 2 tbsp

2 garlic cloves, peeled and minced

4 small chilies, unseeded and chopped

2 stalks of lemongrass, chopped

Coriander leaves, 3 tbsp

Lemon wedges, for serving

Chili powder, 1 tsp

Maple syrup, 1 tsp

Beef broth, 500ml

Kelp noodles, 100g

Directions

Blend chilies, lemongrass, ginger and garlic in a food processor and form a smooth paste.

Heat coconut oil in a large pan and cook the paste for 5 minutes.

Add beef cubes, maple syrup and broth and stir.

Cover the pan and heat the mixture for 1 hour over small flame.

Uncover the pan and cook for another 10 minutes.

Meanwhile boil noodles and drain well.

Put these noodles in a large bowl.

Pour the beef stew over noodles and fold.

Squeeze lemon juice over it and enjoy.

Servings

2 persons

Preparation Time

1 hour 20 minutes

Nutritional Facts

Calories	Carbs	Fat	Protein
502	35g	20g	35g

Thai Turkey Parcels

How about starting your day with low carbs turkey cutlets? These baked turkey parcels not only taste divine but are also extremely healthy!

Ingredients

Turkey breast, 4g finely diced

1 red chili, unseeded and chopped

1 stalk of lemongrass, chopped

1 bunch of coriander leaves, finely chopped

Lemon juice, 1 lime

2 large garlic cloves, peeled and minced

Fish sauce, 3 tbsp

Stir fried Paleo vegetables (of your choice), 300g

Directions

Preheat the grill over medium flame.

Mince turkey fillet in a food processor.

Add coriander, chili, lemon grass and fish sauce and blend again.

Put the mixture in a large bowl and add pepper.

Divide the mixture into 8 small portions and form patties.

Grill these patties for 5 minutes (each side).

Meanwhile, boil noodles and drain well.

Add stir fried vegetables to the noodles.

Enjoy with turkey patties.

Servings

4 persons

Preparation Time

25 minutes

Nutritional Facts

Calories	Carbs	Fat	Protein
173	14g	2g	27g

Paleo-Thai Lunch Recipes

The light and easy-to-cook recipe is not only healthy but also has a divine taste. If you are a chicken lover then try this recipe!

Shredded Chicken

Ingredients

1 fresh ginger, finely sliced

2 chicken breast pieces, skinless and steamed

1 large lemon, for serving

2 shallots, finely chopped

Lemon grass, finely chopped

1 red chili, finely sliced

Thai basil, 1 bunch

Sea alt according to taste

Mint leaves, roughly picked

Directions

Ina pan, add water salt, chili, shallots and ginger and heat over small flame.

Meanwhile finely shred the cooked chicken.

When the mixture starts simmering, add shredded chicken to the mixture.

Turn off the flame when the chicken is thoroughly cooked.

Drain additional water.

Enjoy with any Paleo sauce.

Servings

4 persons

Preparation Time

35 minutes

Nutritional Facts

Calories	Carbs	Fat	Protein
214	6g	11g	23g

Aroma Lobster

Sea-food lovers must try this recipe. If you want to enjoy low-fat sea food diet then this recipe can meet your needs.

Ingredients

1 small sized shallot, finely chopped

20 Lobsters, raw

1 lime zest, grated

Lime juice, 2 tbsp

4 large garlic cloves, peeled and minced

1 red chili, finely chopped

Mint leaves, handful finely chopped

Lemon grass, roughly picked

Coriander leaves, handful

Coconut oil, 100ml

Ginger root, 2 cm peeled and minced

Directions

In a bowl mix all the ingredients except lobsters.

Set aside this paste for 30 minutes.

Meanwhile peel the skin off lobsters.

Marinate lobsters with the paste.

Barbecue for 45 minutes and enjoy with lime zest.

Servings

4 persons

Preparation Time

1 hour

Nutritional Facts

Calories	Carbs	Fat	Protein
137	10g	8g	16g

Cashew Fried Chicken

The unique blend of cashew paste and sizzling sauces is perfect for the days when you are running out of time. You can prepare this dish with very few ingredients.

Ingredients

Coconut oil, 1 tbsp

Unsalted cashew, 1 cup

1 large onion, roughly chopped

1 large mushroom, quartered

1 yellow pepper, finely chopped

1 squash, finely chopped

Fish sauce, 3 tbsp

4 chicken breast pieces, skinless and cut into square chunks

Chicken broth, ½ cup

Maple syrup, 1 tbsp

Garlic paste, 1 tsp

Directions

In a pan shallow fry onion and yellow pepper.

Add fish sauce and chicken broth to onions and heat.

When the mixture starts shimmering, add chicken pieces and mushrooms.

Cook until tender.

Dish out the chicken and serve with cashews.

Servings

4 persons

Preparation Time

30 minutes

Nutritional Facts

Calories	Carbs	Fat	Protein
369	26g	16g	34g

Spicy Shrimp

Another easy-to-cook and healthy recipe for sea-for lovers that needs only few spicy ingredients and stir fried cabbages.

Ingredients

Coconut oil, 2 1/2 tbsp

Fish sauce, 1 tbsp

Distilled water, 1/2 cup

1 cup cabbage, shredded

Finely chopped onion, 2 tbsp

8 shrimps, fresh and peeled

Minced garlic, 1 tbsp

Red pepper, 2 tsp crushed

Directions

In a skillet heat coconut oil and add cabbage to it.

Heat for less than a minute and remove stir fried cabbage from the skillet.

Add shrimps and garlic to the remaining oil and fry until tender.

Add remaining ingredients to shrimps and continue heating for 1 minute.

Pour the shrimp sauce over cabbage and enjoy.

Servings

1 person

Preparation Time

35 minutes

Nutritional Facts

Calories	Carbs	Fat	Protein
406	12g	35.6g	13g

Frilled Chicken with Paleo Dipping

Nothing can be more divine than crispy chicken, dipped into sizzling Paleo sauce! Try this easy recipe and know another side of Thai cuisine

Ingredients

Coconut oil, 2 tbsp

Basil leaves 1 small bunch

2 large garlic cloves, chopped

Chopped onions, 1 cup

2 peppers, freshly grounded

1 cup mushrooms

Boneless chicken, 1 pound

Paleo fish sauce, 5 tbsp

Raw honey, 1 tsp

Sea salt, 1 tsp

Directions

In a medium pan, heat over small flame.

Stir fry garlic and peppers.

Add chicken, honey and salt.

Cook until tender.

Add fish sauce to chicken and stir.

Toss mushrooms and onions and cook for 2 minutes.

Season with lemon juice and enjoy.

Servings

4 persons

Preparation Time

30 minutes

Nutritional Facts

Calories	Carbs	Fat	Protein
244	12g	10g	30g

Coconut Curried Chicken

Coconut curry is a unique dipping and extremely low fat. Try this recipe if you are calorie conscious and sick of boring diet plans

Ingredients

Distilled water, 1 quart

Fresh pineapple chunks, 1 cup

Red curry, ½ cup

1 green pepper

Coconut milk, 2 cans

Maple syrup, ¼ cup

2 pieces boneless chicken breast pieces

Fish sauce, 3 tbsp

Directions

In a bowl whisk curry and coconut milk together.

Transfer this whisked mixture to a pan and heat over small flame.

Add remaining ingredients to the mixture except chicken pieces and mix well.

When the mixture starts shimmering, add chicken pieces and cook well for 15 minutes.

Enjoy with fish sauce dipping.

Servings

6 persons

Preparation Time

50 minutes

Nutritional Facts

Calories	Carbs	Fat	Protein
623	77.5g	34.5g	20.3g

Steamed Thai Mussels

The unique combination of coconut milk and mussels gives a mouthwatering taste to sea-food and is very healthy

Ingredients

Fresh mussels, 5 pounds

Chopped cilantro, 2 cups

Lime juice, ½ cup

Paleo fish sauce, 1 tbsp

Coconut milk, 1 can

Minced garlic, 2 tbsp

Thai curry, 2 tbsp

Directions

In a large bowl, mix coconut milk, curry, lime juice and fish sauce together.

Heat the mixture and bring it to boil.

At this point add mussels and cover the pan.

Cook for 10 minutes.

Remove from flame and enjoy with lime juice.

Servings

6 persons

Preparation Time

30 minutes

Nutritional Facts

Calories	Carbs	Fat	Protein
484	22.4g	24.5g	49.3g

Cashew Butter Kelp Noodles

Kelp noodles are completely Paleo and when folded with Cashew butter, become totally irresistible!

Ingredients

Grass fed butter, ½ cup

Cashew paste, ¼ cup

Finely chopped cilantro leaves, 3 tsp

Distilled water, ½ cup

Kelp noodles, 12 ounces

Fish sauce, 1 tbsp

Coconut oil, 1 tsp

1 large garlic clove, minced

Whipped coconut milk, 1/3 cup

Directions

Mix cashew paste and butter together in a small bowl.

Add hot water to this mixture and mix well until combined.

Add fish sauce, coconut oil, whisked milk and garlic paste.

Prepare Kelp noodles.

Add drained noodles to the mixture and fold.

Garnish with cilantro leaves and enjoy.

Servings

4 persons

Preparation Time

20 minutes

Nutritional Facts

Calories	Carbs	Fat	Protein
580	70.2g	27g	20g

Fried Crabs

Crispy crabs fried in coconut oils cab serve the purpose of perfect lunch on days when your are running out of time

Ingredients

Distilled water, 1 ½ cup

1 large lemon, sliced

Coconut oil, 3 tbsp

1 cucumber, chopped

2 onions, roughly chopped

3 spring onions, finely chopped

3 garlic cloves, finely chopped

Sea salt, 2 tsp

Crab meat, ½ pound

1 egg, whisked

Directions

In a large pan, heat coconut oil over small flame.

Stir fry onion and garlic.

Add water and salt to the mixture and heat for 5 minutes.

Add egg to the mixture and bring the mixture to boil.

Add crabmeat to the mixture and heat for 5 minutes.

Dish out the curried crab and enjoy with cucumber.

Servings

4 persons

Preparation Time

55 minutes

Nutritional Facts

Calories	Carbs	Fat	Protein
304	38g	13g	11.6g

Thai Fish Bites

Fish folded in grass fed eggs is a perfect dish for those who want to shed extra pounds but can't stick to diet plans

Ingredients

Coconut oil, for frying

Boneless fish fillets, 1 ½ pound

1 egg

Coconut flour, ½ cup

4 spring onions, finely chopped

Fish sauce, 2 tbsp

Cilantro leaves, ½ cup finely chopped

Raw honey, 1 tsp

Directions

In a bowl combine, coconut flour, fish sauce, honey cilantro and onions.

Coat fish to the mixture.

In a food processor add fish and egg and blend.

Refrigerate minced fish for 30 minutes.

Form small patties.

Stir fry and enjoy.

Servings

8 persons

Preparation Time

1 hour

Nutritional Facts

Calories	Carbs	Fat	Protein
164	12g	7g	13g

Paleo-Thai Dinner Recipes

Thai BBQ Chicken

Ingredients

3 large garlic cloves, minced

6 skinless chicken breast pieces

Ginger root, 2 tbsp minced

Maple syrup, 1 tbsp

1 lime zest

Fish sauce, ¼ cup

Fresh lime juice, 2 tbsp

Distilled water, ½ cup

Red pepper, ½ tbsp crushed

Directions

Combine garlic paste, fish sauce, ginger root and red pepper in a bowl.

Coat chicken in the mixture and leave for 24 hours.

For barbecue preheat grill and grease with oil.

Grill the marinated chicken for 8 minutes.

Season with lime juice and enjoy!

Servings

6 persons

Preparation Time

1 hour 30 minutes

Nutritional Facts

Calories	Carbs	Fat	Protein
400	50g	15g	20g

Steamed Crab Legs

Ingredients

Coconut oil, 2 tbsp

Crab legs, 2 pounds

3 large garlic cloves, minced

Sea salt, according to taste

Ginger root, 1 inch

Fish sauce, 2 tbsp

Lemon grass, 1 stalk

Directions

In a large pan heat garlic, lemon grass and garlic.

Add fish sauce to the mixture.

Stir for five minutes.

Add crab legs to the mixture and cover the lid.

Heat for 10 minutes.

Sprinkle sea salt and mix well.

Remove from flame and enjoy.

Servings

2 persons

Preparation Time

30 minutes

Nutritional Facts

Calories	Carbs	Fat	Protein
585	5.3g	25g	90g

Grilled Prawns with Sour Cashew Sauce

Ingredients

Lemon grass, ½ cup minced

Sea salt, to taste

Minced ginger root, ¼ cup

Minced garlic, ½ tsp

Fresh cilantro, ½ tbsp

Fish sauce, 2 tsp

Large shrimp, 2 pounds

Lime zest, 3 tbsp grated

Coconut oil, ½ cup

Lime juice, ½ cup

Directions

Add all the ingredients to a large skillet and heat over small flame.

Toss shrimps to the mixture and heat for 30 minutes.

Meanwhile preheat the grill.

Grill the marinated shrimp over small flame.

Enjoy with fish sauce.

Servings

8 persons

Preparation Time

1 hour 30 minutes

Nutritional Facts

Calories	Carbs	Fat	Protein
550	15.1g	40g	30g

Fried Tilapia

Ingredients

1 tilapia, 10 ounce scaled

Chopped cilantro, ½ cup

Coconut oil, 1 quart

Thai basil leaves, ½ cup roughly chopped

5 large garlic cloves, minced

Fish sauce, 2 tbsp

Directions

In a pan heat coconut oil over small flame.

Deep fry scaled fish for 10 minutes.

In another pan, stir fry garlic cloves, fish sauce and cilantro leaves.

Add deep fried fish t the mixture and stir fly for 5 minutes.

Enjoy with fresh lime juice

Servings

4 persons

Preparation Time

35 minutes

Nutritional Facts

Calories	Carbs	Fat	Protein
368	9.2g	30.1g	16.6g

Thai Mild Beef

Ingredients

Kelp noodles, 1 packet

Cabbage, 3 cups finely chopped

Fish sauce, ½ cup

1 large onion, finely chopped

Grounded ginger, ½ tsp

Grass fed butter, 1 small pack

Coconut oil, 4 tsp

Sliced mushrooms, 1 cup

Beef steak, 1 pound

Directions

Cut beef steaks diagonally.

In a large bowl pour salted water.

Heat the water and bring the water to boil.

Add Kelp noodles to the water and cook for 5 minutes.

Drain the additional water.

Add fish sauce, lime zest and grounded ginger to the noodles.

In a pan, heat coconut oil and stir fry beef steaks until tender.

Toss mushrooms and cabbages.

Add noodles to steaks and combine well.

Servings

4 persons

Preparation Time

45 minutes

Nutritional Facts

Calories	Carbs	Fat	Protein
506	79g	13.5g	24g

Pork lettuce Wraps

Ingredients

Pork, 2 pounds grounded

10 lettuce leaves

1 small onion, finely chopped

Fish sauce, 2 tbsp

Tomato paste, 2 tbsp

Lime juice, 4 tbsp

Distilled water, ½ cup

Directions

In a large pan, cook grounded pork until tender.

Add onion and cook for another four minutes

Add tomato paste and stir.

Add water if needed.

Add rest of the ingredients and cook for 5 minutes.

Enjoy with Kelp noodles.

Servings

4 persons

Preparation Time

30 minutes

Nutritional Facts

Calories	Carbs	Fat	Protein
425	12.5g	33.3g	27.1g

Sweet and Sour Vegetables

Ingredients

Raw honey, 3 tbsp

½ pineapple, diced into chunks

Lime juice, 3 tbsp

Fish sauce, 1 tbsp

1 tomato, diced

Coconut oil, 2 tbsp

1 cucumber, sliced

3 large garlic cloves, minced

1 carrot, diced

1 onion, roughly chopped

Directions

In a small pan, add raw honey, fish sauce and lime juice and heat over small flame.

Bring the mixture to simmer.

In a skillet, heat coconut oil and stir fry garlic.

Add onion and toss other vegetables.

Stir fry for 10 minutes.

Pour sauce over vegetables and mix well.

Serve hot.

Servings

4 persons

Preparation Time

40 minutes

Nutritional Facts

Calories	Carbs	Fat	Protein
231	38.7g	7.5g	6g

Mushroom Curry

Ingredients

Coconut milk, 2 ½ cups

Fish sauce, 1 tbsp

Sea salt, 2 tsp

Fresh lime juice, ½ cup

Fresh mushrooms, ½ pounds

Lime leaves, roughly torn

Freshly grounded pepper, to taste

Directions

In a pan, heat coconut milk and bring it to boil.

Add salt and pepper and bring it to simmer.

Add mushrooms and cook for 7 minutes.

Pour the mixture in a bowl and add lime juice to it.

Add fish sauce and mix well.

Enjoy!

Servings

4 persons

Preparation Time

40 minutes

Nutritional Facts

Calories	Carbs	Fat	Protein
261	11.8g	24.4g	5g

Pineapple Chicken Curry

Ingredients

Distilled water, 1 quart

1 pineapple, diced

Curry paste, ½ cup

1 small onion, finely chopped

Coconut milk, 2 cans

Green pepper, finely chopped

Skinless chicken breasts, 2 pieces

Fish sauce, 3 tbsp

Raw honey, ¼ cup

Directions

In a large bowl whisk coconut milk.

Add curry paste and blend well.

Heat the mixture and bring and add chicken pieces, honey and dish sauce.

Bring the mixture to boil.

Cook for 10 minutes.

Remove from flame and toss with pineapple.

Servings

6 persons

Preparation Time

50 minutes

Nutritional Facts

Calories	Carbs	Fat	Protein
623	77.5g	34.5g	20.3g

Paleo Chicken Satay

Ingredients

Grass fed butter, 2 tbsp

Skinless chicken breasts, 6 pieces

Lemon juice, ½ cup

Freshly grounded pepper, to taste

Fish sauce, ½ cup

Curry paste, 2 tbsp

Raw honey, 1 tbsp

Directions

In a bowl, mix all the ingredients except chicken.

Marinade chicken with the paste and leave for 2 hours.

Preheat the grill.

Grill chicken for 5 minutes and enjoy.

Servings

12 persons

Preparation Time

2 hours

Nutritional Facts

Calories	Carbs	Fat	Protein
162	4.1g	3g	28.8g

Paleo-Thai Desert Recipes

Thai Coconut Ice Cream Ingredients

Ingredients

Coconut milk, 300 ml

Fresh mint, handful

1 coconut, dried and fresh

Maple syrup, 90g

Directions

Heat coconut milk over small flame and dissolve maple syrup.

Remove from flame and set aside.

Add grated coconut and mint leaves.

Stir and let the mixture cool.

Refrigerate for 1 hour.

Servings

6 persons

Preparation Time

1 hour 10 minutes

Nutritional Facts

Calories	Carbs	Fat	Protein
300	31g	18g	4g

Thai Iced Tea

Ingredients

Sea salt, 1 tsp

Coconut milk, for serving

Thai tea leaves, 1 cup

Raw honey, ¾ cup

Directions

In a large pan, add distilled water and bring it to boil.

Add teas leaves and honey.

Combine the mixture well.

Remove from flame and add coconut milk.

Refrigerate for 35 minutes.

Enjoy!

Servings

3 persons

Preparation Time

40 minutes

Nutritional Facts

Calories	Carbs	Fat	Protein
180	19g	11g	2g

Coconut Macrons

Ingredients

2 gg whites

Coconut flakes, 7 oz

Raw honey, ½ cup

Sea salt, a pinch

Lime juice, 2 tbsp

Directions

Preheat oven to 280 degrees.

In a large bowl whisk eggs whites and add honey, salt and lime juice.

Fold coconut flakes in the mixture.

Bake for 20 minutes and enjoy.

Servings

8 persons

Preparation Time

1 hour

Nutritional Facts

Calories	Carbs	Fat	Protein
170	26g	7g	2g

Fried Bananas

Ingredients

10 large bananas

Sea salt, 1 tbsp

Coconut oil, 2 cups

Dried and shredded coconut, ½ cup

Raw honey, 2 tbsp

Directions

Preheat oven for 300 degrees.

In a small bowl, mix coconut raw honey and sea salt.

Add a little water and form a thick batter.

Fold bananas into batter and bake for 20 minutes.

Note: You can also stir fry coated bananas.

Servings

20 persons

Preparation Time

35 minutes

Nutritional Facts

Calories	Carbs	Fat	Protein
330	15g	33g	1g

Mango Pudding

Ingredients

Distilled water, 1 ½ cup

Sea salt, 1 tsp

4 mangoes, peeled and diced

Raw honey, 1 cup

Coconut milk, 2 cups

Directions

In a large bowl, pour coconut milk and heat over small flame.

When the milk starts thickening, add honey and salt and stir well.

Mean while, combine magi chunks and water in a food processor and blend.

Add the mango puree to coconut milk and stir for 10 minutes.

Refrigerate for 30 minutes.

Enjoy!

Servings

4 persons

Preparation Time

1 hour

Nutritional Facts

Calories	Carbs	Fat	Protein
150	33g	18g	4g

Paleo-Thai Smoothies

Pineapple-Coconut Smoothie

Ingredients

Pineapple, 2 cups diced into large chunks

Dried coconut, 2 cups shredded

Crushed ice, 2 cups

Coconut Milk, 1 cup

Directions

Blend all the ingredients together.

Enjoy.

Servings

2 persons

Preparation Time

10 minutes

Nutritional Facts

Calories	Carbs	Fat	Protein
270	63g	3.5g	3g

Thai Watermelon Smoothie

Ingredients

Watermelon, 4 cups seedless

Crushed ice, 2 cups

Coconut milk, 1 cup

Lime juice, 1 cup fresh

Directions

Blend all the ingredients together until smooth.

Enjoy

Note: To sweeten you can add a pinch of honey

Servings

4 persons

Preparation Time

10 minutes

Nutritional Facts

Calories	Carbs	Fat	Protein
51.2	13.3g	2g	1g

Ginger Smoothie

Ingredients

Grounded Ginger, 1 tsp

Coconut milk, ¾ cups

Raw honey, 1 tbsp

Fresh pineapple, 2 cups large chunks

Directions

Combine all ingredients well.

Blend until smooth and enjoy chilled.

Servings

6 persons

Preparation Time

5 minutes

Nutritional Facts

Calories	Carbs	Fat	Protein
66.1	15g	3g	1g

Thai Mango Smoothie

Ingredients

Maple syrup, 5 tbsp

Coconut milk, 2 cups

3 large mangoes, diced roughly

Crushed ice, 2 cups

Directions

In a food processor, blend all ingredients together.

Enjoy chilled.

Servings

2 persons

Preparation Time

10 minutes

Nutritional Facts

Calories	Carbs	Fat	Protein
100.9	25g	10g	5g

Ingredients

Crushed and Dried coconut, 16 ounces

Coconut milk, ½ cup

Crushed Ice,

Sea Salt, a pinch

Maple syrup, 2 tbsp

Directions

Blend all the ingredients together.

Enjoy!

Servings

2 persons

Preparation Time

10 minutes

Nutritional Facts

Calories	Carbs	Fat	Protein
50	14g	3g	1g

Paleo-Thai Snacks

Thai Noodles Salad

Noodles with crispy vegetables can serve the purpose of healthy and low carbs snacks.

Ingredients

Shrimps (cooked, peeled and roughly chopped), 2 lbs

4 paleo buns

2 large garlic cloves, peeled and minced

Cilantro, ½ cup finely chopped

1 small shallot, peeled and chopped

Grass fed butter, 1 tbsp

Fish sauce, 2 tbsp

Coconut milk, ½ cup

Raw honey or maple syrup, 2 tbsp

Diced carrot 1 cup

For Paleo Buns

4 grass fed eggs

Coconut flour, 3 tbsp

Sea salt, a pinch

Coconut oil, 3 tbsp

Baking powder, 1 tbsp

Directions

For Paleo Buns

Preheat the oven to 360oF.

Mean while, mix coconut flour, sea salt and baking powder together.

In another bowl whisk eggs and add coconut oil.

Mix the dry and wet mixture together and fold until combined well.

Pour the batter into a flat baking tray and bake for 10 minutes.

For Shrimp Patties

Mince shrimps and form patties.

Refrigerate for 30 minutes.

In a large pan, heat coconut oil, fish sauce, maple syrup together.

Keep stirring until the mixture becomes thick.

Set aside and let it cool.

Fry the patties over small flame.

Sandwich the shrimp patties in Paleo buns and pour coconut sauce.

Servings

4 persons

Preparation Time

1 hour

Nutritional Facts

Calories	Carbs	Fat	Protein
500	34g	22g	44g

Light Shrimp Burgers

Shrimp burgers with crispy spring onions cannot be enjoyed as snacks only, but you can also enjoy these burgers in breakfast or lunch.

Ingredients

Peeled shrimp, 2 lbs large piece

Paleo buns, 4 small pieces

Finely minced garlic, 2 large cloves

Coconut oil, 2 ½ tbsp

Jalapeno pepper, finely minced and seeded

Fresh lemon juice, 2 tbsp

Cilantro, 6 ½ tbsp

Sea salt, 1 tsp

2 large Green onions, finely diced

For Paleo Buns

4 eggs

Coconut flour, 3 tbsp

Sea salt, a pinch

Coconut oil, 3 tbsp

Baking powder, 1 tbsp

For Crumbs

Almond/coconut flour, ½ cup

Coconut flakes, ½ cup finely crushed

Sea salt, 1 tbsp

Lemon zest, 1 tsp

Garlic powder, 1 tsp

Pepper, 1 tbsp

Directions

For Paleo Buns

Preheat the oven to 360°F.

Mean while, mix coconut flour, sea salt and baking powder together.

In another bowl whisk eggs and add coconut oil.

Mix the dry and wet mixture together and fold until combined well.

Pour the batter into a flat baking tray and bake for 10 minutes.

For Filling

Mix all the ingredients of crumbs in a bowl and set aside.

Separate 1/3 lbs of shrimp and mince it in a food processor to form a paste.

Add the remaining shrimp and finely chop it.

Add garlic cloves, cilantro, chopped onions and pepper and mix all the ingredients well.

Transfer the mixture in a bowl, and add crumbs mixture to it.

Combine all the ingredients well and divide it into four equal portions.

Make small balls and flatten gently with finger tips.

Refrigerate.

In a small bowl, mix meshed tomatoes with lime juice.

Add salt and pepper and set aside.

Grease small pan with coconut oil, and heat Paleo buns.

Add more oil and shallow fry shrimp patties.

Sandwich between buns, dress with sauce and enjoy!

Servings

4 persons

Preparation Time

20 minutes

Nutritional Facts

Calories	Carbs	Fat	Protein
479	33g	19g	43g

Thai Eggs Delight

This is a unique Thai snack which is not only rich in protein but also very delicious!

Ingredients

8 eggs, hard boiled and peeled

Distilled water, 4 tbsp

Maple syrup or raw honey, ¼ cup

Coconut oil, ¼ cup

Fish sauce, ½ cup

Freshly grounded black pepper, 2 tsp

1 cilantro leaf, for garnishing

Directions

In a small pan shallow fry finely chopped shallots until they turn golden brown.

Dish them out and in the same pan add a little coconut oil and heat hard boiled eggs.

When the exterior starts turning brown dish out the eggs and slice them in half.

Add fish sauce, maple syrup and water to the remaining oil and heat.

Sprinkle salt and pepper and mix well.

Pour the mixture over fried boiled eggs and garnish with cilantro leaf.

Servings

4 persons

Preparation Time

40 minutes

Nutritional Facts

Calories	Carbs	Fat	Protein
390	33g	23g	15g

Thai Tuna Salad

This unique fish salad can also be served as a side dish. You need very few ingredients to make this salad!

Ingredients

Fish sauce, ½ cup

Fresh basil, 1 cup

Lemon juice, ½ cup

Handful of cilantro leaves, finely chopped

Raw honey, 2 tbsp

1 small fresh black pepper, grounded

Tuna, 2 ½ lbs

1 small spring onion, green and white part chopped

Directions

In pan heat fish sauce, lime juice and honey.

When the mixture starts simmering turn off the flame and pours this mixture over tuna.

Refrigerate for 1 hour.

Take out the tuna and keep at room temperature for few minutes.

In a pan, heat coconut oil for few minutes and cook tuna for few minutes, until softened.

Enjoy with fish sauce and spring onions

Servings

8 persons

Preparation Time

35 minutes

Nutritional Facts

Calories	Carbs	Fat	Protein
246	10.7g	8.4g	31.6g

Final Word

Paleo diet consists of only organic elements (naturally existing food products) and is considered as one of the healthiest ways to shed extra pounds. Thai dishes, on the other hands, are famous for their unique taste all around the world. This report includes 50 recipes through which you can enjoy Thai dishes in a *Paleo* way.

Try these easy and delicious recipes and live healthy!

www.ingramcontent.com/pod-product-compliance
Lightning Source LLC
Chambersburg PA
CBHW080429290526
45791CB00008BA/2435